Look Your Best

A Guide to Style and Proper Dressing for Women

Lisa Lewis

PUBLISHED BY:

Lisa Lewis

Copyright © 2012

Table of Contents

Chapter 1: Introduction

What is the Purpose of This Book?

These days, strict dress codes do not rule our everyday style. Sometimes, it might be difficult for modern women to know, what to wear and when. "To break the rules, you need to know them first." as the saying goes.

This book will help you to understand the etiquette around clothing, and hopefully will generate new ideas. Read this book and be ensured that you, the reader, do not need a doctorate to understand the ins and outs of fashion.

Do you feel confident in your ability to recognize fashion trends? We will go through some key aspects of what it means to be a trendsetter. Most important part is to be inspired by all things aesthetic and keep a keen eye on the fashion around you.

Haute couture designers are partly responsible for the hot trends and fashion, but even they are inspired by the everyday aesthetics, past fashion eras, films and artists that we, mere mortals, also have access to.

Are you aware of fashion trends? Do you want to be among the first to try them? Even so, all latest trends and fashions don't necessarily equal style in modern times. Classics always come first.

Think of Chanel and other fashion icons. They don't change according to every latest whim on the market. What's important is defining your own style and building up a wardrobe that will not go out of style. Everything you buy has to suit you and accentuate your best features.

Anyone can become a stylish and chic individual. Why not be that special woman, who turns around heads everywhere she goes? Some might ask if it is important to be well dressed. Naturally, the paparazzi will not follow you around the clock unless you are a mega-celebrity.

Gardening does not require full on designer wear, but if you show up to corporate events or job interviews in shaggy jeans and t-shirt, your professional credibility might be at stake. Another example: would you want people to your wedding dressed up in bikinis and flip-flops? (Unless it's a beach wedding, I'm assuming the answer is no.)

In the first part of the book, we will go through the history of fashion and offer ideas where to get inspiration from. The second part offers more hands-on advice regarding occasions, clothes and accessories, and hopefully informs you, the reader, of how to dress up accordingly.

Chapter 2: Women's Fashion Through Times

Fashion industry borrows its latest trends almost always from past decades – it could be some statement details, patterns, fabrics, styles associated with a certain era. As a stylish individual, it is handy to know the ins and outs of fashion of the past before creating new, groundbreaking styles for yourself.

There are lots of good books written about the history of fashion. Why not browse through it in your local library, for instance? One such recommended item is *A History of Fashion in the 20th Century* edited by

Gertrud Lehnert. With its beautiful illustrations, this concise manual helps readers to understand the trends of the twentieth century.

Here, we go through some of the highlights of the past and suggest when and where ideas from the previous decades could be used.

The Beginning of 20th Century

The two decades before roaring twenties and its flapper girls could be described as the period where haute couture – high fashion – began. Before 20th century, regulations about who could wear what, where and when were extremely tight and unforgiving. According to *A History of Fashion*, "fashion begins when people take pleasure in dressing up."

What, then, is this haute couture, or high fashion? On one hand, it is an elite form of fashion that was in high demand up until 1960s. During this decade ready-made clothes became more widely available and popular.

We see haute couture design on catwalks, fashion magazines and in advertising, but only a few can afford or have the interest in buying haute couture. Haute couture designer must employ a certain amount of dressmakers, show two collections a year containing a precise amount of new designs and all the designs must be made by hand and to measure.

Fashion and the world changed dramatically in the beginning of the twentieth century. *A History of Fashion* gives an example relating to the length of skirts. Up until 1900s, hemlines always reached down, whereas during the 20th century skirt length has varied enormously. Think of the period costume dramas on television and what the royal women wear. It is hard to determine what period is under scope if you only look at the hemline.

Also, body's natural shape was being emphasized and freedom of movement in clothing came about – whereas before, it was laced up and hidden under tons and tons of material. Again, think of the costume dramas in television – not a lot of skin was revealed and the clothing by rule was tremendous in size.

Another crucial example listed in *A History of Fashion* is the fact that women began wearing men's clothes for the first time. Take for instance flat shoes, trousers and suit jackets – all supposedly unfit fashion items for women prior to 1900s. These days we do not think twice about throwing on a suit jacket, but there was a specific time and place in history where the gender distinctions were challenged.

One key change in fashion was banishment of the corset. Waist less gowns and tunics that were gathered beneath bosom and fell straight into the floor were highly popular in the beginning of the century when small waist was emphasized.

High quality materials, such as velvet, silk, fine muslins were in high demand. Also exotic and orientalist influences – or Western interpretations of oriental – gathered momentum, not only in fashion but in theater, interior design, painting, architecture and so forth. World War I had little effect on menswear, but womenswear became instantly more functional and slimmer silhouettes and shorter skirts appeared.

Roaring Twenties and Flappers

The period between 1920 and 1930 is paradoxical. On one hand, enormous amounts of wealth were being accumulated. On the other, mass unemployment, radical political changes and inflation affected almost everyone. The cultural atmosphere and psychological aftermath of the Word War I was, however, change in attitude. People wanted to enjoy themselves again and be entertained. Variety shows, early cinema and jazz music were evolving and became instantly popular.

As beauty ideals of the day favored boyish figures, slim lines and long legs, fashions borrowed perhaps work best on women who are not all that curvaceous and fairly androgynous. Take note of the flappers if you wish to elongate your legs, for instance. Curvaceous figure was replaced with narrow hips and small bosom. In fact, androgyny in style and dress became fashionable. Fashionable girl of the twenties was boyish. This can be seen in hairstyle, ideal body shape and fashionable clothing.

Consequently, in 1920s one-piece dresses that hid bust and hip were fashionable. Silhouette was straight and squarish, hemline rose to knee, waist line fell to hip and seamed stockings were in fashion.

In evening wear, the most dramatic difference to day wear was the amount of skin revealed. Hemlines were often uneven, and dresses made of sheer, flowing fabric. Decolletage in evening wear was a must. Evening dresses also tended to have more lavish fabric, gold and silver embroidery, sequins, feathers, and fringes. Suits were influenced by menswear, and suits had severe cuts. Trousers, however, were not worn in public yet.

There are particular accessories listed in *A History of Fashion* that mark the twenties, and without obtaining some, no 1920s look is complete. Take for example an eye catching fan, small hats that complemented the short, bob haircuts. In evening wear, no hats were worn but feathers, diamonds, or aigrette plumes were attached to head. Whereas the hair and clothing were simple, straight lined and functional, make up was elaborate and vamp-like.

1930s – 1940s

By the beginning of 1930s, women's hair and skirts became longer again. Boyish, sporty fashion of the 1920s gave way to a more elegant, feminine look. Squarish, angular lines popular in the previous decade became old-fashioned, and more flowing lines began appearing in women's fashion. The new feminine look took inspiration from 19th century role models, women who were delicate flowers, women of leisure, women of indulgence. Bodices were low-cut and often strapless.

Once again, the waist was emphasized, hats became more elaborate and artistic, hair was long enough to be waved and put up. Women's looks became more feminine. Cinema and female stars on silver screen did not only represent fashion and costumes, but also partly helped to create new trends and fashion.

Skirts covered knees and were often calf-length. Tops were narrow, and sleeves small. Bosom was ideally bigger again. For the new ideal shape, women once again began wearing corsets that emphasized the new beauty ideals.

In day wear, skirt and blouse combination was the essential outfit. A bolero could be added, or a suit jacket, that was longer and fitted at waist. In the afternoon and evening a dress was more appropriate than suit.

In practice, this meant wasp waists, full, ankle or calf-length skirts, tight tops, narrow shoulders and padded hips. Masses of fabric were needed, and materials became more splendid than in years. In terms of accessories, hats and gloves made a return. The whole outfit had to be thought out from head to toe. Matching shoes and purses were a must.

Suits were generally the popular day wear 'uniform', but in the postwar period they consisted of tight-fitted skirts that stretched to calf. Jackets were fitted and hip-length. Jacket could be exchanged with matching cardigan or a sweater. Strapless dresses were only seen in evening wear. Daytime dresses particularly in summer were sleeveless, and neckline was low-cut.

1950s – Rock'N'Roll and the Birth of Teenage Culture

In the 1950s, the younger generation began rebelling against the older generation, and in the United States, Elvis Presley and rock 'n' roll music had influence on the youth of the day. Musical icons influenced their fans with their peculiar and particular clothing styles.

Rock 'n' rollers wore glittering, colorful costumes that juxtaposed with the serious suits men were expected to wear prior to 1950s. Movie industry once again influenced the popular culture generally and fashion particularly. For example, James Dean in *Rebel Without Cause* became iconic.

According to A History of Fashion, "adolescence was no longer simply a dominant phase in the life of an individual, but an important factor in society as a whole. The adolescent society of which we speak today has its origins in the affluent society of the 1950s and in the protest of the young rebels of that decade."

Jeans is the number one fashion item of the 1950s. They were worn as leisure wear in America as early as 1930s, but they were imported to Europe in 1950s and became more prominent casual wear. Jeans carry with them ideas of freedom, American lifestyle, and youthfulness.

Denim jeans have become such a household item representing the casual and freedom, that nowadays when you see an invitation with casual dress code, you instantly think of jeans first. There are varieties of jeans on the market and it can be a puzzle to decide what jeans fit you the most. See the subsequent chapter on jeans for further information on how to choose your own killer jeans.

1960s – Swinging London and Summer of Love

1960s was a decade where radical changes in political, social and economic levels took place. Key changes consisted of sexual liberation and identity politics. Beauty ideals changed as well: the new iconic female was a child-woman, like Twiggy, and to be young and sexy at any cost was crucial.

Patterns and dress lines changed to balloon shapes, tent dresses and A-line dresses. The dresses of the 1960s didn't include any decorative details, refined cuts, and were cut from stiff, synthetic fabrics. Great colorful graphic or floral patterns made them statement dresses. Hairstyles varied from backcombed to simple bobs.

Both women and men went barefoot, grew long hair, wore elaborate jewelry and jeans and shirts in colorful patterns. Long, flowing flowery dresses and flowers in hair were also popular among women. Rustic, old-fashioned blouses became popular, as well as native styles and other items borrowed from past eras.

Street fashion as a concept was born in the 1960s. It was no longer the elite of fashion houses or strictly designers who determined what the latest trends were. Instead, the styles of the ordinary youth that became popular dominated the fashion world. Great Britain and particularly swinging London was the trendsetter in 1960s. So when thinking about great 1960s looks, the Beatles and other Brit invasion bands come to mind. Mod culture was trendy, and women of the time aspired to look like the famous model Twiggy, for instance.

Carnaby Street in London was the place, where the 'in-crowd' and sharp looking 'mods' shopped either in boutiques or second hand stores. Second hand and vintage was first popularized right there and then. These days, strolling down the Carnaby Street is a bit likes walking down the memory lane. However, cool vintage shops and funky second hand stores are to be found everywhere.

1970s – Back to Simpler Times

In 1970s, natural elements and handmade items were popular in interior design, furniture and fashion. Knitwear suddenly became fashionable again. Patchwork items were considered romantic and reminded of simpler, happier times. Indeed, nostalgia and ethnic styles ruled the fashion discourse of the day. The beauty ideals respected naturalness in all aspects.

For instance, the so-called grandma shirts, long peasant skirts, gypsy skirts and Indian shawls were popular items in women's fashion in the 1970s. It was important to mix and match elements from different cultures and traditions, and the outcome was often colorful and eccentric.

All in all, 1970s style was more informal and casual than before. Even the evening wear aimed for casualness rather than elaborate elegance. Midi and maxi skirts – calf- or floor-length – were highly popular as opposed to the mini-dresses of 1960s. Coats were often this length too, and underneath them, women wore contrasting miniskirts or mini shorts. Fur-lined coats and jackets often included a hood, borrowed from sportswear. Here we have another nod towards highly casual clothing.

Pantsuits for women became also popular day wear and arguably socially acceptable for the first time. Pants were meant to hang from hips and they widened towards the flare. Bell bottoms like these compliment most body shapes and make both men and women appear slimmer.

1980s & 1990s

1980s as a cultural period is marked by idealization of success and achievement. Fashion in this decade had become international, playful and postmodern in character. As in the previous decade, 1980s fashion borrowed from the past, but this was rather a 'remix' than 'replay', to borrow terminology from music.

Empire lines, high waists and neoclassical draping were one thing copied and transformed, as were the puffy sleeves and tight vests from 16th century, hippie fashion from two decades before was manipulated into something new. This all has happened in haute couture. Everyday fashion looked different. Co-existence of different styles and trends was acceptable; there needn't be a definite style for everyone. This is one such ideological fashion statement that women nowadays should keep in mind. There's simply no need to be fashionable at the cost of one's own style.

Sportswear and sporty clothing became one variation of daytime wear, whereas glamor ruled evening wear. Also day wear sported a look 'dress for success' for women. Career women preferred suits at office hours, long wide blazers with broad shoulders, often heavily padded, worn with a slim line skirt and heels. A powerful woman in such clothing was seen for example in Dallas and Dynasty, immensely popular soap TV series of the 1980s.

As with previous fin de siècle-generations, 1990s also awaited the end of century and millenia with mixed feelings. Revivals of earlier styles continued as in the eighties. Youth fashion borrowed from 1960s and 1970s, whereas for example John Galliano's haute couture moved to 1920s. In parallel to 1970s revival, a new style called grunge is born. Floral dresses are combined with heavy duty boots, and the new female is eclectic. Techno music, MTV and new technology inspire mix matched, futuristic looks.

The division between fashion and non-fashion becomes blurry. What emerges in the nineties is the brand and the label and their importance. Whereas in 1980s wealth was made into a parade, in 1990s it is all about understatement and small detail, such as the label, that reveals fashion sense and wealth.

As always, latest fashions recycle old, well-proved trends from the past. A number of sub-cultures also exist that mix and match elements from the bygones. Think for yourself here – what could be taken from the past that flatters you? What are you interested in? What looks do you need to obtain and keep in your wardrobe? Some current trends and clothing can be disposed quite quickly, but all women should hold on to such classic items as the cocktail dress.

For great inspired looks from the past, look at the TV series, magazines, pop stars of the day. Makeup and hair tutorial videos can be found from YouTube for authentic looks. Flea markets, thrift stores and vintage stores offer good selection of clothing and accessories, and don't be afraid of mixing roaring twenties with for example eighties style.

Ebay and other online auction houses are also full of authentic vintage wear in all price ranges. Happy bidding! If there is a little seamstress in you, you could order vintage patterns again from Ebay or other online auctions and make your own clothes. In the next chapter, we will go through some further sources of inspiration both in print and online.

Chapter 3: Inspiration

Where to Find Inspiration from?

Individual dress style does not happen overnight. Most stores and boutiques offer advice and tips when requested, but it is not very chic to buy complete outfits straight off the mannequins in shop windows.

Besides, since the globalization has ensured, chain high street brands like Swedish H&M, Spanish Zara, American Urban Outfitters and Spanish Mango are almost everywhere, one needs a little imagination to stand out.

Inspiration is everywhere around you. Have a cup of coffee in a café, sit by the window and watch the world go by. Style on the streets can be very inspiring, keep a keen eye out on stylish people about you. What are the women in such popular TV series as Sex and The City wearing?

Affordable versions of their designer wardrobes can be found, and new points of views of mixing and matching items and accessories are presented in every episode. Do not wrinkle your nose at following haute couture designers – it need not be deemed as an elite practice. Most haute couture designers and fashion houses are not aiming to produce functional, every day dresses. However, their artistic collections shape what will become trendy in high street stores.

There are other outlets for inspiration that you can pool in from the comfort of your own home. Fashion magazines and blogs offer valuable insight and new ideas. Why not also research some past fashion icons to help determine your own, individualistic and stylish look.

Fashion Magazines

When talking about fashion magazines, one particular publication comes to everyone's mind – regardless of how committed they are about style and womenswear. This magazine is Vogue. It was first published in the United States in 1892, and since then has spread globally. There exist a number of national variations of Vogue – most notably France, United Kingdom, and Italy.

Vogue has been described in *The New York Times* as the most influential fashion magazine on market. What makes Vogue so special, then? American Vogue's editor, Anna Wintour, is acknowledged to be behind her magazine's success. She took over as a chief-editor in 1988, and since then has become a style icon herself with her trendy bob haircut and sun glasses she apparently never removes.

Wintour allegedly has enough power and influence in the clothing industry to make or break an upcoming fashion designer. If an interest has sparked in you to find out more about what goes on behind the scenes at Vogue, why not rent out the critically acclaimed and hugely popular film *The September Issue* that documents Vogue in the making. Vogue can be read in print or online at www.vogue.com

Other popular fashion publications include for instance Cosmopolitan, which does not strictly contain fashion editorial and articles but also spreads on general women's lifestyle. Cosmopolitan does offer editorials on latest trends and for example very helpful shopping guides, but can be overwhelmingly sexual in other content at times. Be warned.

Harper's Bazaar is another publication worth familiarizing with. This magazine is available in print and online at www.harpersbazaar.com, and as Cosmopolitan, it also contains material on relationship and love in addition to beauty, hair style and fashion tips. According to some, Harper's Bazaar is a bit more elegant, sophisticated and artistic than most women's magazines.

Fashion Blogs

Fashion blogs are another great way of snooping around for astonishing trends, exciting news and great tips. The blogosphere seems full of fashionistas making their own mark on industry. The content varies.

There are so-called 'shopping blogs' where the blogger typically demonstrates with words and pictures what they have bought and from where. Following these blogs can be extremely helpful, because when you spot something that is eye-catching you will be immediately informed where the item is available and in what price.

Some fashion bloggers are actually aspiring photographers who upload their experiments with fashion shoots. Third group of bloggers fall into a more general category, where typically fashion, trends, styles and all things aesthetic are commented and shared with the readership.

Browsing through the so-called amateur blogs is a good place to start for what is fresh and up-coming in the market, but there are a few established and well-seasoned bloggers that are highly recommended.

One such is Susie Bubble's www.stylebubble.co.uk. "Susanna Lau, also known as Susie Bubble, is a writer and editor living and working in London. Lau started her blog 'Style Bubble' in March 2006. It consists of her widely read thoughts, personal experiences and observations on fashion with a focus on spotlighting young and unknown talent."

London has always been the hotbed for upcoming and groundbreaking fashion, and in the recent years the center of style, aspiration and hip has moved from Carnaby Street to the old working-class neighborhoods of East London.

True East End fashion spirit can be back traced by looking at /www.whatkatiewore.com/. Here is a blog, where a couple in marketing made a name for themselves. The gist was that Katie wore a different outfit every day, and her boyfriend captivated outfits on film and wrote editorials in form of love letters. It does not get more romantic than this, ladies.

Here's an idea: why not start your own blog to record your experiments in style and latest acquisitions made. The point is not to aim for a Pulitzer Prize on your journalistic achievement, but to receive feedback from followers and readers and to interactively engage with other, perhaps more experienced, trendsetters.

Fashion Icons

Fashion icons are celebrities that leave a mark on the public not only with their professional attributes, but by their characteristic fashion sense and sometimes groundbreaking fashion choices.

They are considered not only jet setters, but trendsetters. These fashion icons normally gain a timeless status, and are seen in classics.

Maybe they even contribute to what is deemed as classic. Looking back at such female figures can help you to understand, what it means to create your own style. We can take tips from all of them, and add a little bit of fashion icons into our own closets and everyday wear.

Coco Chanel – or, Gabrielle Bonheur Chanel by full name – was born in Paris at the end of 19th century. In 1910, she established her own fashion house at the age of twenty-seven. Her career in fashion began with designing hats that became the talk of the day. She then extended her business into sportswear and womenswear which were received with great enthusiasm.

Some of the Chanel classics include the Chanel no 5 perfume, the stitched, black handbag and the elegant, simple suits. Chanel is also the name behind the very first 'little black dress', or cocktail dress.

Coco Chanel herself dressed immaculately and many people consider her a style icon. Chanel believed in luxury, but not in flashy ornaments or overstatements. Simple elegance is her signature look both in private life and in designer business.

How to dress like Coco Chanel, then? One key aspect featured on almost all writings about Chanel's personal style is the use of contrasting colors, black or navy-blue and white, with architectural proportions. The little black dress and matching shoes and bag are also 'musts' when imitating Chanel style.

Marilyn Monroe – or Norma Jean Baker by birth – was born in 1926 and died in 1962. Her premature death was one contributing factor in her cult persona. Marilyn's career began in modeling, and soon enough her captivating appearance was recognized by studio executives at 20th Century Fox.

She appeared in around 30 films and is most remembered for her light, comedic roles as a blonde bombshell, but also delivered flawless roles in more serious representations, as for example in her last role in *The Misfits.*

Marilyn provides another example of elegance and glamor, but with emphasis on different elements. In her hay day, the beauty ideals expected more feminine and sumptuous looks from women.

At the height of her career in the 1950s, women aspired to have hour-glass figure, hair was ideally long and wavy and the style of clothing feminine. Marilyn was the epitome of all that.

Marilyn – like Coco Chanel – was not a woman of added-on flash or overstatements. According to some style experts, her wardrobe was based on dresses – even so, she managed to look radiant in ordinary jeans. Perhaps the secrets to her ultra feminine look was the carefully considered colors (she looked good both in bright and pastels), high heels and elegant jewelry such as pearls.

Audrey Hepburn was born in Belgium in 1929. She experienced a lot of changes in scenery in her early life, as pre-war she lived both in England and Holland. After the World War II, she moved to London to study ballet. Like Marilyn, Hepburn also modeled before being spotted by film producers. She appeared in thirty-one films and died in 1993.

Audrey Hepburn is probably most remembered for her role as Holly Golightly in *Breakfast at Tiffany's.* In this film, she wore a remarkably stylish and yet overtly simple sleeveless little black dress in the style of Coco Chanel.

After starring in *Roman Holiday* and sporting a white, plain blouse, she caused this item to become extremely fashionable. See now why all fashionistas ought to follow films as well as catwalks?

All in all, Hepburn was a delicate figure and her choices in clothes and accessories reflected and emphasized her body shape. We will discuss bringing out our best elements with clothes a tad later. Other key items that all Audrey-wannabes ought to have in stock are capri pants, flat shoes, boat neck tops, elegant neck scarfs and top it all with large, dark sunglasses.

Mary Quant is a style icon born in England in 1934. She gained success as a fashion designer, like her French counterpart Chanel. Quant opened her own boutique on King's Road in 1955, and expanded her business into Mary Quant-chain in 1963. She is allegedly the inventor of miniskirt, and a forerunner of the so-called Chelsea Look.

Mary Quant's iconic style can be attributed to the daring miniskirt and the sharply cut geometric hairstyle. This bob was cut and designed by Vidal Sassoon and could be called the 5 point cut.

1970s fashion icons include Farrah Fawcett, Debbie Harry, Bianca Jagger, Liza Minnelli, Olivia Newton-John, Anjelica Huston, Jane Fonda, Patti Smith and Pam Grier amongst others. We will focus on the style of Farrah Fawcett here since she seems to hold some crucial qualities typical to the 1970s looks in general.

Farrah Fawcett was born in the United States in 1947, and spring to fame in 1970s as Jill Munroe in *The Charlie's Angels* that was a hugely popular TV series of the time. She is considered as the sex symbol of the 1970s and her dress sense should be studied for the authentic 70s effect.

Basically, Fawcett's style begins with the iconic hair do, 'feathered shag' – a wild, bleached but natural looking flow of hair. She often wore flared denim jeans, which makes her an ultimate dress icon to be kept in mind when thinking about casual wear.

Fawcett's evening looks were typical of seventies – glamor, gold-plated, shiny and flashy. Evening dresses in Fawcett's style ought to be maxi-length and seemingly flow. Sleeves can be long, or dresses sleeveless.

Vivienne Westwood is another British fashion designer that has left her mark in the world of fashion also with her personal style. She was born in England in 1941, and Westwood first sold her clothes in a shop called Sex, and they were seen on the infamous punk band Sex Pistols. Her first collection Pirate was seen on catwalk in 1981. She has influenced the provocative punk style, and is a very colorful personality.

What can we learn from Westwood herself? Some of the provocative and colorful items seen on Westwood are a bit 'too much' on as ordinary folks and mere mortals, but perhaps the lesson here is to try out different styles and items without prejudice. All of us need courage to dress up individually. Breaking rules are not something to worry about.

Westwood's punk style and ideology can be broken down to such items as classic Doctor Marten's shoes, punky jewelry that perhaps carries a message to the public, different patterns mixed up ruthlessly, outstanding colors and fearlessly unconventional pattern cuts.

Westwood can be compared to such recent pop stars and fashion icons as Lady Gaga. Perhaps either of these two don't carry such items that we could furnish our own wardrobes with, but nevertheless, their influence and sporting of design can help us to determine our own aesthetics.

There are a few key items to attain Madonna's famous 80s style. Begin with a good pair of leggings worn under a short skirt or denim jeans shorts. Black tank top or a t-shirt with a slogan makes a good top, and a lace bustier was often seen on Madonna as a top, not an undergarment. As for shoes, ankle boots will do. Accessorize with lace gloves, bangle bracelets and a multitude of necklaces – for example religious ones.

Chapter 4: Looking Your Best – Body Shapes, Color Schemes & Little Tricks

In this chapter, we will go through the basic body shape categories that most women fall into. One type of fit, silhouette or pattern does not suit everyone – so how should you know what accentuates your type best? Not to worry, we have the answers right here.

Additionally, we will look at color palates and skin tones. Unfortunately, your favorite colors might not bring the best out of you. The good news is that we have the tips that will help you fill your wardrobe with flattering colors.

Is there anything I can do to make my legs look longer, you might wonder. We have some suggestions here that might help you out, whether it is longer legs or slimmer waist you're after. Clothing should not feel uncomfortable on you, and one of the magical aspects of fashion is the fact how much you can change your appearances with simple tricks of the eye.

What Body Types are There?

It's time to get down with the business. One of the first practical things to do when renewing wardrobe is to find out what body types are you, and to know what does not suit you under any circumstances. See if any Gok Wan programs are on re-run on TV – he is a master of suiting and booting women of different shapes and figures.

For our purposes here, body shapes can be divided into rectangular, hourglass, apple, strawberry and pear. Obviously, people in actual life cannot be categorized thus. We all have different physical attributes, and it takes a trained eye to determine what we really want to bring out and what to fade out, retrospectively.

If you find it hard to see for yourself what fits you, or unable to make educated guesses at department stores, find a member of staff or an in-house stylist for a second opinion.

Rectangular body shape means a person who could use more curves, ideally. Rectangular ladies are pretty straight up and down, from shoulders to hips. Hour glass shaped women have well defined bust and hips, while the waist is slimmer.

Apple types carry typically more weight around their waist, while pear types have emphasized lower sections of the body. Hips and bottom can be problematic for pear types. Strawberry shaped ladies generally have broad shoulders and/or big bosom, which bring out the upper body.

The key idea behind body shapes and dressing accordingly is to bring out your best bits in proportion. Numerous guides and tips are available online, but Joy of Clothes' Shape Guides are highly recommended for further reading at www.joyofclothes.com/style-advice/shape-guides.

What Suits Rectangular Women?

Rectangular women's priority is crafting an illusion of a waist. Rectangular women should keep silhouette free of clutter, and focus on details on hip and bottom area. Women of this body type should not wear clothing with noticeable waistbands or high-waisted items.

Straight lines do not compliment rectangular ladies, as they do not accentuate waistline at all. Boxy jackets and double breasted coats and jackets ought to be dismissed completely if you fall into the rectangular category. As for sleeves, ideally a stylish rectangular woman sports loose fit, puffed, flared, rolled up or ¾ length sleeves. Neckline options are lower and wider lines, like scoop boat.

Rectangular shape should go for simple and clean style lines when it comes to tops and shirts. Opt for items that are round at necklines and/or sleeves. Empire lines and tops that drape under chest work miracles for rectangular women.

Jackets ideally are structured, and as with tops, round necklines should be looked for. Coats are no exception in the straight line rule – additionally, some emphasis on the waist could be added.

Rectangular women could try for example kaftans with splits at waist. Other dress styles that compliment these figures are simple, straight lines, empire and shift dresses. When it comes to trousers, rectangular shaped have variety of choices.

Why not opt for low-waisted options that have flare or wide leg. Boot cut is also not only acceptable, but recommended for this body type. This goes for jeans as well. Embellishments and details on back pockets work great.

Joy of Clothes' Shape Guide offers advice about swim wear too. Soft cup bra in swimsuits and form fitting waists are encouraged, as are two piece options. Bikinis are thus allowed for rectangular types. Colors should be fairly outstanding and bold, plunging necklines apparently make bust and bottom stand out. If you opt for one piece swimsuit, avoid one color and choose perhaps a swimsuit with a stripe at waist line.

All in all, rectangular women's first priority is to emphasize waist. Think of the flowing, feminine lines of the 1940s and 1950s when you put together a killer outfit. Thin belts at that time were used to accentuate and highlight the waist area. Low-cut options work better on the bottom of the outfit.

Best Looks on Hour-Glass Body Shape

Hour-glass type has long been a beauty ideal when it comes to body shapes, but careful consideration on what lines and fits to wear applies to hour-glass women as well. Shaped and fitted items that follow hour-glass body line works best, but volume around curves should be avoided, advises Joy of Clothes' Shape Guide.

It is elementary to wear a supporting bra that will lift the bust and define the waist. Shoulders and necklines ought to be emphasized – try for example scoop, square or sweetheart necklines.

Wider and lower necklines accentuate the center of hour-glass body. Hiding waist with straight lines is not an option; neither are high-waisted bottoms. High necklines or narrowing leg lines will not bring attention to the right areas.

When it comes to tops and shirts, shoulder pads could be effective. Joy of Clothes' Shape Guide recommends cross over tops or wraps, and fabrics ought to be soft. Empire line works well for hour-glass types too. Jackets and coats, as everything else, should be fitted and single breasted. Wide lapels are preferred.

Dresses that fit hour-glass shape best include wrap or shifts, and empire lines. Note that hemline should reach knee level – unfortunately miniskirts will not bring the best out of hour-glass shaped girls. Pencil skirts, however, work fine and compliment the figure.

In jeans and trouser area, hour-glass ladies do best with such classics as boot cut. Straight leg line is most effective, whereas narrowing legs and skinny jeans can be problematic and not fit well the sumptuous hour-glass body.

Again, hour-glass ladies could take in tips from the 1930s, 1940s and 1950s when beauty ideals favored women with ample waists and full bosom and bottom areas. Long, flowing lines and silhouettes work best for hour-glass shape, as do any accessories or cuts that highlight the waist.

What Should Apple Ladies Wear?

Details around bust, tummy and hips should be avoided where possible. Lower part of the body can be as detailed as you wish. Joy of Clothes' Shape Guide advises apple ladies to purchase straight lined or slightly fitted clothing, choosing softer fabrics means that bulk will not clutter your bosom, waist and tummy, and shoulders however, do need attention.

Apple-shaped women should avoid at all costs belts that only worsen the body shape. This means belts of all sizes. Sleeves should exceed your bust-line, when you have your arms by your body. Details and volume should be kept to minimum near the problematic areas, bust, tummy and hip.

As opposed to hour-glass ladies, apple-women ought to wear skirts that rise above knee level. This is good news, as apple-shaped ones have the chance to show off their legs with for example miniskirts, A-line dresses or shift dresses that feature hemlines ranging from mini-mini to knee-length.

Tops and shirts that fit apple-women feature simple lines, empire lines work wonders. A well-fitted bra is also a must on apple-women's check list. Jackets ought to be of single button that can be placed under your bust and above tummy.

Other option is to wear jackets open. Coat of an apple lady can be a-line or cardigan style, and again worn open. Lapels should be relatively big and shoulder pads are strongly advised. Sleeves should be ¾ length or above the wrist.

A-line dresses look best on apple ladies and attention should be diverted from the tummy area. Most flattering skirts that apple shaped women can have are also A-lined, panelled and side fastened. Think of Twiggy, Mary Quant and mod ladies of the 1960s.

Not that all apple ladies should go for the psychedelic, flower power patterns and looks, but take a look at the quintessential A-line and shift dress period. These cuts are the ones that work wonderfully on apple-shaped body.

Darker colors are recommended for apple shapes, at least when it comes to jeans and trousers. Ladies with additional weight around their midsection ought to keep it simple in the bottom half of the body – jeans and trousers should not be fussy. Apple women should also note that flat fronted trousers with wide legs are more flattering than for example skinny jeans.

Right Type of Clothing for Pear Shapes

Ladies who represent the pear shape should ideally balance their top half with lower half, and this effect could be achieved with clothing that makes shoulders stand out and seem broader. Joy of Clothes' Shape Guide advises pear women to wear jackets and tops that either exceed the widest point of hips and bottoms, or finishes just above them.

Pear women should go for layers, volume, clutter, patterns or color on their top half. According to Joy of Clothes' Shape Guide, this creates visual interest and the eye naturally seeks out the upper half of the body. This way, an illusion of sleeker hips, bottom and thighs is created. Waist should be emphasized with for fitted styles.

Pear-shapes ought to avoid creases in leg line, narrowing leg, pinstripe suits, turn-up trousers or wide and flared leg lines. Joy of Clothes' Shape Guide also recommends that pear ladies stay away from combat or cropped trousers. Belts on hips and details that draw the eye downwards around hip area should be avoided where possible.

When it comes to tops, dresses and skirts, hemline shouldn't finish on the hip or thighs, because this again draws the attention to the problematic areas. So that's no miniskirts for pear-shaped ones. Dropped waistlines also tend not to accentuate pear-shaped ladies' best bits.

What about necklines and sleeves, then? Pear-shaped women ought to invest in wider collar and lapels, and to go for boat and bardot necklines. Sleeves can be ¾ length, or puffed and either short or above wrist.

Tops and shirts should be fitted, and particularly recommended are wrap tops or empire lines for pear shaped ladies. Vests, waistcoats and stiff fabrics are also a good way of complimenting the right areas. Shoulder enhancing shapes like shoulder pads, shawls, boleros, wide straps and boat necks all work wonders on pear shaped bodies.

As with tops, jackets should also feature details, collars and perhaps pockets. Trench coats that highlight shoulder area work very well indeed. Fitted shapes and belts are well-worth considering.

What kind of trousers and jeans should pear shaped women opt for? Joy of Clothes' Shape Guide states that dark boot cut denim is best when it comes to jeans. Trousers ought to be plain, as all the 'fuss' should generate attention to the top half of the body. Trousers ought to be bootleg or flared, and simple styles are preferred. As for length, best effect comes out of full leg line or ankle length.

Recommendations for Strawberry-Shaped Women

According to Joy of Clothes' Shape Guide, strawberry ladies ought to go with clothing on bottoms that give the illusion of broader hips. Details and volume should be strictly on strawberry's lower half. Top ought to be clean and uncluttered, and silhouette brought out with dress lines. Accessories such as wide belts create the illusion of a waist, and are highly recommended for ladies with broader tops.

Strawberry types should avoid anything that emphasizes their top half of the body, and items that make them appear broader on top. A few necklines that are out of the question for strawberry-types are for example, boat and bardot lines. Big straps and collars are also a big 'no-no'.

Shoulder pads, puff sleeves and scarves around neck are also details that bring the attention to your top half, so strawberry ladies ought to approach them with caution, if at all. Hemlines shouldn't narrow, because this again highlights top half of the body and thus pencil skirts and skinny jeans should be left hanging on the rail at department stores.

Joy of Clothes' Shape Guide offers detailed advice on what to wear in case you are strawberry type. As to tops, simple straight lines or wrap tops are encouraged. Anything that brings out the waistline works fine, so consider splits on the waist or hips, and layering on hips. Jackets and coats, along with tops, should be straight lines.

Jackets can be flared in hemlines, for example. Coats shouldn't feature strong, eye-catching collars, and in general coats are recommended to be either constructed or shaped with angular lines. Hip pockets and vents in the back should work great for strawberry shaped ones.

Dresses too should follow simple straight lines, but shifts and A-lines work wonderfully. Details like pleats and perhaps even strong patterns compliment strawberry shape. Skirts should have dropped waistlines. Length of the hemline can be anything between short and flared to maxi dresses.

Trousers and jeans should have styles that highlight bottom and leg line. Consider baggy or combat trousers, embellishments on back pockets, flares and wide legs. As for jeans, boyfriend style is recommended.

Boyfriend style refers to any ready-made items that look as if they are modified from men's wear lines. Boyfriend jeans are the opposite of skinny jeans; they are loosely fit and comfortable. Boot cut jeans with flared leg are a safe choice for this body shape.

Color Schemes – How to Know What Colors Accentuate You the Most?

Aside the shape and size of your body, you ought to also consider what colors bring out the best in you. This may mean that your favorite colors are not the most suited after all, and a trained eye of a stylist, make-up artist, or a salesperson at department stores could give you valuable insight.

Women's Day periodical is available in print and online at http://womansday.ninemsn.com.au. According to their article 'How to Choose Which Colors Suit You Best', perfect color combinations can revitalize your look and even make you appear younger. Hence, it is very important to determine not only what to wear, but in what colors.

Best colors for you make you look fresh, elegant and young. Determining your color palate will depend on your eye color, hair color and the tone of your skin. Watch yourself in the mirror and observe your skin tone. Best result for this process is achieved under natural light.

Can you detect a hint of golden undertones, or perhaps apricot? If so, you are of warm toned. In case you detect pinkish hews, you are cool toned. If you belong to the latter category, opt for the colors based on blue. Warm toned women look their best in yellow-based colors.

Warm toned women suit natural, earth colors. Pick out items that are brown, bronze and sage green. Peach and apricot work for example in the summer time. Out of the red scale, warm toned women should choose brick red, dark tomato or burnt orange. These tones accentuate and compliment your natural skin tone.

Also, olive, jade and other earthy greens enhance warm skin tones. Clean ivory or oyster whites compliment with juxtaposed warm skin tones. When choosing business attire, remain with clothing in taupe or bright navy. Brown and gold accessories are highly recommended, as these help you to get out the maximum impact.

Cool skin tones can be enhanced with pure white, deep greens, royal blue, raspberry pink, plum and black. When it comes to red shades, ruby red is an excellent choice. Additionally, cool skin tones can be matched with soft pastels, like baby-blue and pink.

Little Tricks

Aside the systematic regime of buying clothing that suits your body shape and accentuates your color palate; you might have other areas in your physique that could use an oomph or a little trick to draw the attention to your best bits.

Longer legs could be one of the things we aspire to. Flapper fashions of the twenties have some key ideas that will help in this. At the time, boyish figures and longer legs were favored over curvaceous figure and feminine looks.

Whether you are a more feminine hour-glass shape or prefer slightly more androgynous looks, longer looking legs can be achieved easily. Perhaps opt for the knee-level hemline and stockings with seams.

These elongate legs and help create the illusion of killer pins. Also, shorter hemline and seamed stockings trick the eye into thinking that the body shape all in all is longer, and the person taller and slimmer.

Twenties fashionable patterns help to accentuate slimmer, boyish bodies and create the illusion of narrower hips and smaller bust. If this is the look you are aiming for, consider elastic corsets, waist line that is dropped to the hip, and perhaps lavish sleeves that balance the basic silhouette.

Do you feel that your waist should be accentuated or do you need an illusion of the waist created? Both of these problems can be solved with proper clothing.

What to wear if you want to emphasize your waist? One such thing is V-neck line when it comes to blouses, shirts, tops and cardigans. It makes your waist appear slender and diverts attention away from the middle section of your body.

Another great look is under-breast cut styles that camouflages the lack of waist. This style means a top or a dress, that has either fabric plaited under breast, or a pattern where there is a separate piece of fabric sewn to create a stripe. For best results, choose items that also have a V-neckline. You could look for plaited tops, dresses, cocktail dresses, evening wear and so forth.

When it comes to jackets and coats, opt for items that mimic the shape you aspire to have. Jackets and coats should have tapering at waist and extend downwards. Consider throwing on a belt to accentuate waist line. When the hemline is longer, or has additional features, an optical illusion of length is created and waistline appears slimmer.

Skirts, on the other hand, should expand on the hips. This again tricks the eye, and your waist appears slimmer. Think for example pencil skirts that can shape the silhouette. The bonus aspect of pencil skirts are the fact that it can be effortlessly worn during the day in the office.

With adding a few festive accessories, pencil skirt transforms into an evening wear easily. Dresses should also expand a little from hips, and should have either cut under breast or V-neckline. If you want to draw the attention away from the waistline, go for tunics or dresses cut off the breasts that extend downwards. Perhaps even opt for loose tops that are gathered about the hips.

You should avoid tops with no shape and loose silhouette. Leave dresses that have no shape at waistline and high neckline to the rack because they will not accentuate waistline and will make the silhouette seemingly shapeless. Coats and jackets without waistlines should be ideally left out from your wardrobe entirely, but add on a belt if needed.

See that there are no pockets around waist, as this will only expand the waistline and make you appear heftier. Short boleros and cardigans that don't expand all the way over the waistline will also make you seem wider at waist.

What about bigger bust? Can an illusion of bigger breasts be achieved with right kind of clothing? Of course, here's few tips how to achieve this look.

Consider buying padded bras: this is the very first step. After that, opt for details or busy patterns around the area you want to enhance. For example, you could wear tops that have slogans right across your breasts.

Another option is wearing sleeveless tops and dresses if the weather permits this. At least during the summer or indoors you can enhance your bust area with going sleeveless. Right neckline also plays an important role in creating the illusion that your bust area is bigger.

In this case, you want to avoid low necklines such as V-necks, as these firstly work to draw attention to other areas and also points out to your bust. During winter or chillier times, high necklines like turtlenecks work wonders.

Accessory wise, opt for long necklaces that accentuate and enhance your bust. Try for example wearing long, bold chains. Chains or pendants should fall past your breasts.

Chapter 5: Key Items

Do you often look at your ram packed wardrobe and feel that you have nothing to wear? Not to worry, this is a common thing. The problem is that instead of focusing on key items and matching clothing we hoard all kinds of items from sales. We don't keep in mind that one piece of clothing can be transformed to serve from one look to another with simple combination tricks and right kinds of accessories.

Here, we go through some key items that every woman should have in their wardrobe. Additionally, we will explain how these items could be transformed and used from dusk till dawn.

Jeans

As a general rule of thumb with all clothing, women should consider what their body shape is and make decisions and purchases based on this information. We have discussed body shapes by large in a previous chapter, but let us talk of jeans in particular here.

Not everyone needs to look like Kate Moss to don jeans. Just remember, that even though particular jeans are fashionable, one cut does not accentuate all.

Low-waisted jeans, like the classic boot cut, make both women and men appear slimmer. This effect is taken further with jeans that are not only boot cut, but have flare or wide leg lines. These kinds of jeans are highly recommended for women, who believe to be perceived as rectangular shapes.

In other words, if you have a straight upper body and perhaps a longer torso opt for boot cut or low waists, paired with flare or wide leg line. These jeans also work wonderfully with women, who have perhaps some additional weight around their tummies. Apple shaped women with extra weight around midsection should also stick to darker colors when it comes to jeans.

Contrary to the common belief, not even women with sumptuous hour-glass figures can pull everything off. Straight leg line and classic boot cut brings out the best of hour-glass shaped ones. Narrowing legs and skinny jeans might not accentuate the hour-glass women.

If you have extra weight around your bum or thighs, attention should not be drawn towards your lower-half of the body. Jeans should be boot cut again, and plain in details. Simple jeans styles are the best for pear shaped ladies. Best effects are created with full leg lines or ankle length jeans.

Boyfriend and baggy jeans work best for women, who have more volume in their upper body. These women have broader shoulders and strong upper bodies. Their jeans ought to highlight bottom, and leg line. This is best accomplished with baggier jeans with flared leg lines.

Vintage jeans are available through the normal vintage clothing routes: online and in second hand shops. There are even stores specializing in vintage jeans. If you already have a pair of jeans that have that retro-look, you could easily make your denim trousers look worn and unique.

This is a great look, always trendy and easily achieved at home. Begin with washing the clothes, and placing them on a suitable workspace. You need to decide how much damage will be done to jeans. Keep in mind that over time these jeans will become increasingly worn, and going over the top with distressing jeans is maybe not the most far sighted option.

Sandpaper could be used in creating a distressed look on brand new jeans. Place a block of wood inside the leg when you are grating or sanding the jeans, so you will not press through the other side of leg by accident. If sanding by hand seems a weary idea on the distresser consider using (carefully) a power sander on the job.

Distress – or artificially age denim – denim with a razor blade. Begin from the edges, and as you wash the fibers of the fabric, it will begin separating. Razor blade or utility knife could be used for this.

You could also make small cuts to the fabric and tear with your hands until the intended level of raggedness is achieved. Knees and thighs are normally the area where jeans get worn, so do the ripping on these areas.

After attacking your jeans with knifes, scissors, sandpaper and power tools, wash the denim once more. All the changes will not necessarily take place immediately, but rather prepare the fabric. The fiber of the denim will start breaking down after the initial wash after distressing.

How to fade your jeans? Aside from the cuts and distressed areas, you ought to consider fading your jeans for that perfect, worn-out look. One way of doing this is to fade your jeans in the sunlight during the summer. Some experts say that once you have washed your jeans with detergent hang them outside in the direct sunlight for roughly two weeks.

However, if you want quicker results you may want to use bleach in the fading process. Work fast, as the bleach damages fabric and ought to be washed off as quickly as possible. Remember to wear gloves to protect your skin from the harmful effects of bleach. Apply the bleach with a sponge and cover the work surface with an old towel, for example. After you have applied bleach in desired areas, wash your jeans separately in cold water.

Cocktail Dress

A little black dress is an evening or cocktail dress that is normally cut simply and hemline is short. It originates from Coco Chanel's early collections of the 1920s, and became popular in the postwar era.

A History of Fashion defines cocktail dress in following words: "more dressy than the afternoon dress, but less formal than an evening gown because it was never floor-length and generally less ornate." Cocktail dress is indeed very versatile and an important part of every woman's wardrobe.

Regardless whether you're witnessing haute couture collection on a catwalk or a high street collection at a department store, you will find a little black number featured in almost all collections.

The trick is to find a timeless, classic cocktail dress that suits your figure and all kinds of occasions. Think Audrey Hepburn in her classic performance as Holly Golightly in *Breakfast at Tiffany's*. She wore the now famous little black dress – or LBD – designed by Hubert Givenchy together with classic pearls.

Perhaps you ought to opt for a little black number that has little detail, is classic cut and could be used in a number of occasions. It shouldn't become dated, so think twice before going for too trendy options.

Cocktail dresses obviously come in many other colors aside black as well, but black is by far the most classic choice and should be obtained before playing around with brighter, funkier colors.

Little black dress is essential for every woman's wardrobe and can be dressed down or up depending on the occasion and event you are attending. During the day time, you can accompany your little black number with ballerinas or bumps and a suit jacket – you will not seem out of place at the office.

More detailed and elaborate accessories like white pearls, fine jewelry and sassier heels are used to dress up your little black number. Your hairdo should be more considered and fancier when wearing the little black dress at evening functions.

Suits

Even if you don't work in a business-minded environment, where business attire is needed, you should own one perfect suit combination: a jacket and matching trousers and a skirt. These items could be mix matched with other items and like little black dress they can be dressed up or down depending on the purpose.

We will talk of business attire and the professional dress code later during the course of this book, but for now, let's focus on the suit that every woman ought to have hanging in their wardrobe.

When shopping for the perfect suit, keep in mind that you are looking for something versatile, classic and flattering. This means that you should stick with a neutral color: black, navy blue, grey and charcoal are all good options. Choosing a neutral color that compliments your color palate ensures that you can use either the jacket or the trousers and skirt with other items, and you needn't worry about color coding.

Secondly, make sure that the suit fits you perfectly. Ill-fitting clothing makes you look sloppy, not sassy and will most likely not accentuate you. The better the fit, the more confident you will look in your 'power suit'. If it helps, consider super heroes or heroines – your suit should fit like their costumes fit them and create the identity.

Having said that suit should fit perfectly, it doesn't mean that you're doomed if you don't find your perfect fit straight from the rail. You may not have the budget to get a suit tailor-made, but alterations cost less than getting the whole suit done from the scratch.

Many high street and department stores also offer affordable alterations services, be it extra length you need to get rid of in leg line or sleeves. Take into consideration the kinds of shoes you will most likely be wearing – heels and flat shoes require different length in leg line.

A smart looking suit skirt should be at least knee-length, but if for example a pencil skirt or calf-length hemline suits you better, go for it. Sleeves should reach wrist and not an inch further. Make sure the jacket accentuates your body shape to the tee.

It is entirely up to you whether you wear your suit jacket with skirt or trousers at work – *if* you wear a business attire to work. Jacket and a skirt combo works at weddings, business occasions, funerals (if you opt for black), where as trousers might fit better at job interviews perhaps.

You could lose the jacket and wear a dressy blouse with the skirt or the trousers at more casual affairs, such as dinner parties. Also, consider throwing on your blazer or suit jacket with jeans, shorts and dresses for a great look on casual affairs.

White Shirt

White dress shirt is a classic that compliments the suit well, but can be worn in a more casual way as well. We found some amazing tips from Chic Fashionista-webpage at http://www.thechicfashionista.com. Here's just a few of them.

In addition to white dress shirts, you could have a few in accentuating colors or perhaps even in stripes. This way, you can alter between days and it will not seem that you are wearing the same outfit every day at the office.

There are a number of ways wearing your white dress shirt outside the corporate environment. For more relaxed – even feminine, perhaps – look, leave the top buttons unbuttoned. This way you'll look and feel less stiff and manly.

Details in white shirts vary. Why not opt for puffed sleeves, pleats and belted waists to get a more personal feel to this key wardrobe item? Keep in mind that you ought to have one simple, classic dress shirt that will not get dated too soon.

As with many of the other key items in every woman's wardrobe, accessorizing your white dress shirt makes a world of difference. How about adding on some statement jewelry, scarves or a belt?

Another bonus side of belts is that the dress shirt can be unfitting, and adding one on will makes the shirt fit from waist. You could wrap the scarf around your neck and let it hang lose, or tuck it under the collar like men's tie. Jewelry could potentially add on color and sophistication. For a more bohemian, eclectic look, hippie-style jewelry works wonders.

White dress shirt could also be worn under a V-neck sweater or a cardigan. This works both at the office and on your free time. Cardigan could be unbuttoned or buttoned up, as long as the shirt itself is unbuttoned at top. Buttoning too much up might make you look less chic casual and more prudent boring.

Another great way of wearing white dress shirt is with a vest. This is a sophisticated look and suitable for office and outdoors – casual dinner party perhaps or for going out in style? Accompany this look with a necklace or a colorful scarf to add extra oomph. Dressy vests are a great option for wearing blazers or suit jackets.

White dress shirt paired with neat jeans also works at many occasions, and those with killer legs might want to pair white dress shirt with jeans shorts at summer. Additionally, add a leather jacket or a classic trench if weather requires a coat.

White dress shirt can also be paired with your 'power suit' skirt or more casual skirts. Pencil skirt with a white dress shirt – always tucked in – is a classic look that is suitable to wear at the office and with added on statement jewelry at a dinner date, even. Those with extra weight around their midsection might want to cover the tuck-in with an appropriately long cardigan.

Accessories: Handbags, Shoes, Scarfs, Jewelry

Buy scarfs that are either bold colored or printed and add oomph to your most basic outfit: jeans and T-shirt, for example.

Flat shoes that are classy enough to wear at office or parties are a must. Ballerinas seem to have secured a place as classics and are widely available in different colors and with differing details. You may want to consider more colorful and funkier flats that can spruce up an outfit easily. Keep in mind that they should fit more than one outfit – versatility is the key when shopping for the essential wardrobe.

Black pumps are also a key item in your wardrobe. You can have as many heels as you like in all available colors of the world, but you'll be lost in the office and outside without black pumps. These heels will never go out of fashion, and can be worn in every occasion, be it weddings, office environment, hot date or a Sunday brunch with the girlies. They will go with all outfits, are versatile, and accentuate all body types.

White pearls – real or fake, it's up to you – will never go out of style and are a must, even though you wouldn't wear them every day while doing grocery shopping. Accompanied with the little black number, the white pearls really come out and this is a perfect, classic look for all kinds of events.

Additionally, you might want to keep some statement jewelry on hand. These could be bracelets, necklaces, rings or earrings. Add these bold accessories, over-the-top to any of your outfits to look more chic and dressed up.

Underwear

Every woman should always have a new pair of panty-hoes available. In addition, you could get some colored or patterned panty-hoes to spice up your more plain outfits. Seamed stockings also make you appear sophisticated and more feminine, and they also make your legs seem longer.

Bras and matching panties should also be kept 'in stock'. Of course, you will need more comfortable granny underwear and sport bras available too. Brassiere should absolutely be well fitted for the maximum effect.

If you need help, lingerie sellers will be happy to help with choosing right kind of support. Some modern women consider slips and undershirts old fashioned, but they still have a clear function. Perhaps, if obtaining these seems too much of a hassle, purchase the slimming, shaping underdress.

Here are just a few classics and essentials. When gathering your functional, dream wardrobe, your needs and hobbies will of course state what you ultimately have to buy. However, these key items can save the day and all outfits can be based around them. Let us spend some time finding out what of these classic pieces you should wear at certain occasions.

Chapter 6: Occasions

How to Dress Up for Different Occasions

The rule of thumb in its most simple, straightforward sense is that there ought to be different wear for day and evening time at least. However, there are varieties of different occasions where the etiquette defines the clothing. These rules are not given or universal, but we will go through some of the most crucial ones.

Some say that it is always better to underdress than be the overstatement in the crowd, but in some events you may well *want* to be the center of the attention and stand in the limelight, perhaps with the aid of your fashion sense. It is important to learn how to play these things by ear.

Casual Business Dress

Long gone are the days when pretty much only men worked outside home, and when the dress code was simple enough – either you were a white-collar or a blue-collar worker. Obviously, white-collars referred to office jobs, where men traditionally wore a white shirt under a suit jacket, tie and suit trousers. Blue-collars, accordingly, meant manual labor and blue uniforms.

Today, however, the situation is entirely different and luckily women at offices and work places have to spend some time planning on the office attire. Start with a pondering session over a cup of coffee, perhaps. What is the message you want to give out to customers and clients? What will your clothing say to colleagues? What is the general dress etiquette at your office?

Again, most of these work place environment codes are not written per se. Probably no one will hand out memos on what to wear next week, so chic ladies once again have to play by ear and observe the world around them. Here we will go through some basic ideas about casual business dress for your convenience.

Standard business attire for ladies consists of suit jacket, which, however, is optional but preferred in senior roles. You can vary your standard business with suit skirt or a skirt that matches the jacket. Skirts should be of darker tone or perhaps beige, but they have to be at least knee-length.

Optionally, you can wear pressed, tailored trousers with creases. Blouse or shirt is normally white. Shoes ought to be closed-toe and low heels, although high heels are not entirely condemned. Coat should be smart as well, and macs or trench coats for example do the trick.

When it comes to business casual, the terrain gets much more complicated. Some people understand 'casual' as jeans and flip-flops, but that might send the wrong message to the work community and clients alike. Play it safe, ladies.

Don't reveal too much skin and stick to the minimum of knee-length when it comes to dresses and skirts. Neutral tones like black, grey and beige are preferred over neon green and the likes, but consider wearing an eye catching statement accessory that could be of a bolder, vivid color.

All sources tell us to avoid logos or slogans we see everyday on people's t-shirts on streets. Classics never fail you – no one has to be a trendsetter at the office. With casual business attire, you could for example switch suit jacket to a cardigan or a pullover.

Still need further reading? Why not visit the ultimate dress code tool online at www.dresscodeguide.com/.

What should you do when you want to mix it up a little bit? Wearing the plain suit with a white dress shirt every day might get a little repetitive. Suit jacket could be exchanged to a cardigan or left out altogether. Different, bold colored scarves could do the trick. Alternate between skirt and trousers, and occasionally wear a dress – perhaps your little black number with the right accessories?

Job Interviews

How to dress to impress for job interviews? Such situations always have great emphasis on the first impressions. Therefore, one should really think out what to wear in order to send the right signals for that potential, future employer. Regardless of the actual work environment, it is a safe bet to dress up professionally for the interview procedure.

Professional interview attire is closely connected to the business attire. Always opt for a black, grey or navy blue suit. Skirt should be approximately knee length. Since the interviews tend to be situations where most people feel a tad uncomfortable or nervous, skirt should be of length where sitting down feels comfortable. All in all, suit should be comfortable but fitting.

Blouse should be coordinated to match the rest of the attire, and white color still dominates the professional attire when it comes to shirts and blouses. You might want to spare those killer heels for hot dates or nights out in clubs and wear flats or more conservative shoes to an interview.

Jewelry should be understated and minimal. Hair should be neat, and go easy on the make-up and perfume. Portfolio or a briefcase is, of course, an essential accessory.

For some interviews, less formal attire is acceptable. Opt for the formal wear if you are unsure of what the environment will be like. Overdressing and going for the more formal is never a bad look at job interviews.

Too casual look, could, however ruin your chances. In informal interviews you have some options for the professional, suited and booted look. See for example what business casual attire includes. In all interviews, tattoos should be covered and piercings kept to earrings.

Corporate Events

How to look sassy and chic while still remaining a convincing professional? Elizabeth Conway offers her advice in the article 'Work Event Dress Codes, Decoded' up on The Daily Muse website. Conway's career has revolved around corporate events and professional functions, so she has pretty good insight into this tricky business.

When it comes to men, the dress codes are pretty straightforward and leave little room for interpretation. 'Casual' for men means they can toss on pretty much anything they desire. If the invitation states that the function is business attire, men will wear a suit either with or without tie. Cocktail parties require suit with tie. In black tie events, men ought to wear tuxedos.

Women's event attire can be broken down into four categories: casual (or no specified dress code), business, cocktail and black tie – mimicking the simple subgroups of men's event fashion. Conway offers comfort: casual is the easy one, ladies! Find out what you're comfortable in, and ensure that your attire is casual and fits the season.

Casual events are perhaps are chance to shine and show who you are outside the office environment. "Just choose something you wouldn't be embarrassed by, if your boss saw you on a Saturday." Conway concludes on casual affairs.

What should you wear to an event, when the dress code is 'business attire'? Timing is of essence here. If the function begins fairly early in the evening, then you ought to opt for something that makes you look like you have just finished a meeting with an important client. This look could come out of a high-waisted pencil skirt or sleek black pants with a tucked-in silk blouse.

If the event starts later, or happens during the weekend, ladies should dress up to something that is a bit more 'cocktail' than 'business'. Wear something that is appropriate for the office, like a traditional black dress and add some oomph in the evening time with statement jewelry and fancier shoes, perhaps. This simple transformation "tricks people into thinking I've had time to change" exclaims Conway.

"It has to be five o'clock somewhere in the world," goes the famous excuse for drinking outside cocktail hour. Cocktail parties and the dress code 'cocktail' are tricky, as they stand in a middle ground between business attire and tuxedos. One key rule is to opt for silk materials and never to choose cotton or cotton blend fabrics.

One way of going about determining what to wear for cocktail parties are to look at the outfit in comparison to work environment and a man in tuxedo. If you wore this attire to office, would it be too fancy?

If you stood next to a man in tuxedo in this dress, would you feel underdressed? When the answers to both of these questions are 'yes', you have hit the nail in the head and are ready to leave for that cocktail party.

All women ought to own at least one non-strapless cocktail dress or little black dress as they are also known as. "You can use bold accessories and fun shoes to give the dress an entirely new look – and wear it over and over, without looking exactly the same." Conway concludes on cocktail look.

Again with black tie events, women could again benefit from imagining a situation, where they stand next to a man in tuxedo. If your attires match in a sense that you do not feel underdressed, then you are good to go.

When it comes to length, the dress can be long, knee length or tea length. By tea length we mean dresses that vary from knee to calf length. Anything above knee simply will not do, and this length ought to be preserved for cocktail and other casual occasions.

If you want to stand out from the crowd, think colors! Men and most women will opt for the classic black, but it is not set in stone that formal attires should be black. "A formal event gives you a great opportunity to distinguish yourself by donning a beautiful color," writes Conway.

At the Beach, By the Pool

What to wear at the beach and by the pool? Well, swimsuits or bikini, d'uh, one might say. It is a bit trickier than that, actually. One thing that determines swimwear is the body shape discussed before.

Life Tools for Women website lends a helping hand at these matters. Juliana Day writes of perfect swimsuits and the importance of acknowledging your body types while choosing swimwear.

Large bust is considered a gift according to some beauty ideals, but overflowing cups can cause an unwanted stir. This problem can be minimized with spaghetti straps or wide straps on swimsuit or bikini. Sports top is also an option worth considering, writes Juliana Day.

Women with small bust, paradoxically, may want to purchase bikini tops with pads in order to get a little curve going on in the chest area. If more coverage is the thing for you, horizontal necklines or bloused tops to give an illusion of more busts are what you need. Apparently this will draw the eye to shoulders and divert attention away from the chest.

Do you have a long torso that stands out? If you feel like your upper body dominates the overall effect you might want to consider options that balance out your appearance. Long torso could be shortened with horizontal stripes on a bikini.

Using stripes allows the eye to focus on the top and bottom instead of the middle section. Sports tops work for women with long torsos. Adversely, women with short torso should go for vertical stripes.

Halter top bikinis and swimsuits accentuate women with wide shoulders. Thick straps help the shoulders to look more in proportion.

Women with a bit of a tummy, for example apple types, might want to draw attention away from the midsection.

This illusion could be created with all-familiar empire lines and empire waist. Juliana Day advises to go for dark, unicolored swimsuits "for a more streamlined look." Why not try on a V neckline? This attracts the eye towards the chest and face.

Pear shaped ladies who have more weight on their hips, thighs and backside could try out a skirt, shorts or a beach wrap around their bottom half. Opt for a bloused top that creates proportion and helps minimizing the problematic area.

What to do if you feel short legged? A high cut leg on swimsuits could help and make your legs appear longer. Shorter ladies perhaps ought to go for one-piece swimsuits, as bikinis break up the body figuratively and causes you to look shorter. Skirts or shorts are a definite 'no-no'.

Casual Dinner Party

One of the easiest occasions dress wise is a casual dinner party. You ought to be more concerned with what wine to bring with you than your attire. Anyway, the attire could consist of a comfortable dress or jeans accompanied by a dressier blouse or top.

The key idea is to mix and match comfortable with dressy elements. Casual does not always mean what you are most comfortable in, but dressing up your every day wear. This effect could be achieved with statement accessories such as pearl necklace, classy shoes or a fancy hand-bag.

The location also weighs in here: is the dinner party at a restaurant, or at a close friend's house? Will the event takes place indoors or perhaps outdoors in a patio? If the party happens outdoors, weather elements should be taken into consideration, but note that a dinner party is an evening affair and thus wearing shorts and flip-flops makes you appear perhaps a tad underdressed.

Weddings

What should guests at wedding wear and what types of wedding affairs are there? Always pay attention to the dress code marked in the invitation and dress accordingly.

Another crucial element that female guest should not under any circumstances are to wear white attires – unless it is clearly specified in the invitation that the guests should wear white. This might be a theme in some weddings, but in any other case white is out of question for guests.

Judith Martin, also known as Miss Manners, has written a helpful guidebook about wedding etiquette. This book is aptly titled Miss Manners Wedding Etiquette and it features advice on dressing up as well as some more general issues.

Miss Manners wonders if modern weddings are becoming to imitate the famous Academy Awards Ceremony. The similarities, according to Miss Manners, include outrageous outfits, red carpet for grand entrances, jokes and teasing from master of ceremonies, rehearsed outpourings of gratitude, acknowledgment of sponsors, and so forth.

What interests us here, of course, is the dress code. Weddings are not the right forum for these 'outrageous outfits'. Also, according to Miss Manners' view on wedding etiquette, attending a wedding ceremony and reception shouldn't be thought of as walking down the red carpet – unless you're the bride.

Wedding etiquette for guests seems a little strict and some may wonder, what is the purpose of it in these modern times. One such explanation may be that this occasion is a social ritual where we gather to witness and celebrate two people forming a union. In effect, we should dress up collectively and according to some basic rules to create a feel of festiveness and of communality.

Unfortunately in many modern weddings, the wedding party itself is not clothed in unison, and none of it matches. Also, the wedding guests' appearance ranges from business suits to jeans.

There are a number of online sources where to get ideas and advice on how to avoid becoming a complete fashion victim at wedding ceremony and receptions. The basics you should consider before choosing a dress from wardrobe or purchasing a new numbers are the level of formality and the time of the day. Will this be an informal or formal wedding? Is it taking place in the afternoon or in the evening?

Business attire is acceptable for weddings taking place in the morning. However, most informal weddings take place in the afternoon or in the evening. During the afternoon, short dress or a suit will do the trick whether it is an informal or formal event.

Black is generally considered unsuitable color for day, but it all depends on how you combine and compliment it. Black dress could be worn underneath a brighter colored jacket, for example. At the other end of the range, sequins and too sparkly items are considered too 'dressy' for daytime and thus, should be avoided.

For informal evening times consider throwing on that famous cocktail dress. Your little black dress could be accessorized to give it a bit more personality. After all, this is not a funeral so it would seem a bit absurd for all the female guests to attend in all-black.

If the invitation specifies the wedding to be a formal evening or black-tie event, female guests should wear long dress or a fancier, dressy cocktail item. Note that black-tie events are those happening after six o'clock in the evening, and the term derives from men's attire. Men wear suits, white shirt and a black tie to these events. They are more formal than for example cocktail, but not as formal as white-tie.

In white-tie events, long gown is a must and additional glamor recommended. For that sassy, chic look you may want to consider real or faux fur or diamonds. Opera-length gloves could be a dressy option here, but remember that these gloves should only be worn with sleeveless or strapless gowns. Gloves should also come off when you are eating or drinking.

Autumn and winter weddings at least in northern hemisphere means that you need to wrap up a bit more than during the summer. If your outfit consists of a fur coat in the evening or a suit jacket during the day, then the problem is solved so to speak.

Suit jacket ought to match the dress – this should go without saying. Before heading to the wedding, take a moment in front of the mirror to evaluate your outfit. Will you look smart and fitted with the jacket on? Later you might want to lose the jacket when heading for the dance floor – is the dress underneath appropriate in its own right?

Shrug or a bolero could be another option for chilly weddings. These will not hide your dress in the same way as suit jacket, but they will keep your upper body warm in the autumn and winter times. A brightly colored shrug or bolero could also add to your outfit, if you considered otherwise wearing your little black dress for the event.

So much for the guests – what if it is your wedding day, and as a bride you are not only responsible for your own dream gown but for the wedding party's appearance as well?

One of the most pleasurable aspects of organizing the wedding is the choosing of your own wedding gown. Regardless of what the wedding etiquette says, this is your day and your chance to be the princess. Essentially, if you please, this is your chance to break the rules and wear the dress of your dreams.

Traditionally wedding dresses are white in color, and the variation has come out of picking up the shade and silhouette. White color in western cultures was made popular by Queen Victoria in 19th century and white color has been seen as a symbol of purity.

In eastern cultures wedding dresses are often times red. Finding the suitable tone of white matching the skin color is important, but white color itself is not set in stone anymore.

Consider with your groom what kind of wedding you are organizing and whether some other color is more appropriate and accentuating to you personally. There is no need to hide your personality when it comes to weddings.

These days, floor length gowns are popular choices, often strapless and accompanied by a veil. This convention could be broken down as well – if your invitations invite tea dresses from the guests, your gown could be mid-calf length as well.

There are a range of accessories to consider too – from tiaras to gloves, from flowers to jewelry, without forgetting that classic veil. Whatever accentuates you best, and whatever you've always dreamed of.

When it comes to dressing up maid of honor or the group of bridesmaids, look no further than Martha Stewart's Weddings website up at www.marthastewartweddings.com. According to Martha Stewart's website, bridesmaids in the days of yore traditionally wore the exact same outfits – the same color and shade, the same dress.

These days, however, a range of options is available for brides and maids alike. Modern brides are advised to let bridesmaids to choose styles and pick colors that suit them. For example, bridesmaids can choose from a variety of necklines that accentuate them best – strapless, halter and sweetheart necklines being some of the festive ones, for instance.

Bridesmaids could wear their own dresses with a specific hue, or why not consider a specific designer range? As Martha Stewart's Wedding website states, "many designers have developed dress lines for just this purpose, so you can get many different cuts in exactly the same shade of pink."

When the bride is making the decision for the bridesmaids, she should consider the body shapes of her bridesmaids and what suits each of them best. Dress silhouettes should accentuate bridesmaids' bodies. Does the bridesmaid army vary in body types? If so, then it is probably best to stick with different dress patterns and shapes for each.

Some styles previously considered unsuitable for weddings, such as short hemlines and strapless bodices, are wholly acceptable these days. Even cocktail dress, the little black number, is gaining popularity, although once upon a time black was a bit of a 'no-no' in female section of the wedding party.

If you opt for the little black dress, the bridesmaids possibly either have one already in their closet or can use the same dress again and again. Bridal dresses these days are beautiful, and not hideous, as Martha Stewart's Wedding site notes. "For the first time in a long time, they're trend-based and style driven." Hence, when picking up bridesmaids' dresses, one quality to evaluate is the re-usability. Would the bridesmaids wear these again? If yes, then we have a winner.

Dress codes traditionally have determined the appropriate outfits for the bridesmaids. However, you have some room for personal preference here. "These days, anything goes: your maids can wear short dresses to a black tie affair, or long ones to a casual outdoor bash."

Consider the fabric in relation to the level of formality and location, though. Cotton fabric would seem out of place in an evening setting, and long taffeta dresses would likewise make your bridesmaids seem overdressed in a garden party.

Formal floor length evening gown could be worn both in white and black tie events. Dressy little black numbers should be reserved for black tie and less formal events, though. White tie requires long gowns from the wedding party.

Proms

Proms is a shortened term for promenade, which is a formal black tie dance organized for high school students. So, in dress code terms, it means a black suit with white shirt and a tie for young men. Young ladies have a variety of options here. This is normally seen as a major event for teenagers and possibly their first touch to formal evening wear.

It is an important night for the youngsters, and the chance to dress to impress in school setting can be an exciting, memorable event. Perhaps modern day proms could be compared to debutante balls of the past, where young ladies were first introduced to the society.

Perhaps the most thorough online guide about proms is the Prom Girl website at www.promgirl.com. It features advice on accessories, dresses and flowers and all things imaginable.

Choosing the right, flattering dress that makes the young lady stand out is of course the most important part. We will begin at going through the wide range of optional accessories here, however. As with other formal events, one should be dressed from head to toe at proms and therefore accessories are not simple trinkets, but important parts of the whole outfit.

Jewelry plays an important part in one's prom night ensemble. Jewelry can complement your dress or gown, and it is a channel to use for self-expression. Right kind of, personal and glittering jewelry can makes one stand out from the crowd. Consider jewelry as a statement.

One key rule regarding formal gown and jewelry, is that you should not wear too much of jewelry at once. Jewelry's function is to accent and enhance. There is a chance that too much jewelry or a wrong kind of piece may overwhelm the look of the dress or the overall style.

Perhaps with such formal events as proms, ladies of all ages might want to play down on the jewelry front. Minimum jewelry is fine with most gowns, so consider wearing only earrings and a necklace. One simply can't go wrong with classic pearls, be they real or dress jewelry.

Excessive jewelry that looks out of place sends out the unwanted message of 'flashiness'. In addition to jewelry, young debutante ladies could choose hair accessories.

Accessories do not always simply accentuate your look but could serve a functional purpose. Weather conditions should be taken into consideration. A sophisticated wrap could be added for extra warmth.

What kind of wraps go with evening gowns? Faux fur is one inexpensive option that adds instantly glamor to prom dresses. Alternatively, you could go for a pretty scarf, suitable shawl or a funky cardigan. Make sure that whatever you wear on top suits and complements your gown.

The finishing touch to that perfect, flattering outfit that either makes or breaks the look is purse. You could opt for a small purse, clutch or a bag. Young ladies do not need to bring in tons of stuff, only a few items are necessary. Hence, the purse should not be big or bulky because it might be uncomfortable to hold on to a grand bag all night.

What about the actual dress, then? First of all, as with any outfits, one needs to determine the body shape. You can only make good, informed decisions, if you know what flatters your figure. Best judgment can be made if the person underneath the clothes is acknowledged. Personality plays just as important role as the body shape.

There are a number of options when it comes to prom dresses. Princess or the A-line dress accentuates some girls better than others, and makes an ideal prom dress. Empire dress with its scooped out, high waist works better on some young ladies.

Hemline can alternate from knee to floor length. Floor length ball gowns, according to Prom Girl webpage, can have either a top fitted at waist or a corset style top, "Both tops work with the Ball Gown's large, billowing skirt," states Prom Girl webpage.

You can either go strapless and/or sleeves, but there is also variation in possible sleeves of the prom dress. Cap sleeves cover the shoulders and upper arms, but reveal rest of the arm and are suitable for toned arms.

Sleeves that puff at the shoulders and narrows down towards the wrists are called Juliet sleeves, and they are a perfectly acceptable and festive option if arms need covering.

If you desire to show off shoulders and neckline, but need some warmth in cooler climate, you may want to purchase and don a wrap. Alternatively, get a dress with sleeves that start below the shoulders.

Traditionally, the young gentlemen purchase the flowers worn at the prom. Both attendants need to have matching flowers, and since it is the gentleman who chooses the flowers, the risk exists that the corsage does not match your dress.

Young ladies are advised to inform their dates what suits their dress and perhaps even accompany the date to the florist. If you do go down the florist together, take a picture of your dress or a sample of the fabric with you. This way, the florist can coordinate your corsages with the chosen dress.

In case you are wearing gown with no straps, consider wearing your flowers at your wrist or perhaps even opt for the handheld – or nosegay – corsage. There are other creative ways of wearing your flowers.

Why not integrate flowers to your hairdo, or pin them to your evening bag? Young ladies could also attach their flowers to ribbons. This could be tied around neck or even such unusual places like around the ankle.

Buying the prom dress straight from the rack at a department means that you might show up to see other girls wearing the same dress. There is also the cost. Seventeen magazine's online version tips its readership off a webpage called Coco Myles at www.cocomyles.com. This is a service provider, that offers custom made bridesmaid dresses, but it could easily be used for prom occasions as well.

This award-winning service allows you to customize your dream evening dress online. You can choose from a range of available necklines, hemlines, fabrics, colors and beading. You could also order a matching shawl or a scarf from Coco Myles.

Alternatively, choose a dress that was inspired by a famous actress in a color that accentuates you. All this cost approximately 200 US dollars and shipping charges, so Coco Myles is definitively a considerable option for those budget-minded young ladies.

Again, EBay and other online auction houses are guaranteed to be jam packed with inexpensive options for glamorous, elegant and chic prom dresses. Browse through your local second hand, vintage and thrift stores – you never know what gems might be hiding in them.

You should note in your calculations that second hand dresses will most likely need altering done by a professional or a skilled sewer. As we already know, elegant look comes from a well-fitted dress.

If you or someone is willing to help you have the skills, perhaps you could opt for making your own prom dress. Homemade dress is guaranteed to be original, personal and custom-made in character. Sewing your own dress also means that the cost stays minimal – all you pay for are the basic supplies and fabric.

It all begins with choosing and purchasing the pattern of the dress. These are available in stores and online. Choosing the right pattern depends a lot on the same factors as choosing that perfect dress – the only difference is that when buying the pattern you have to imagine the dress on you.

Most trusted and popular sewing pattern brands are Butterick, Kwik, Sew, McCalls, Simplicity and Vogue. There, also exists a number of sewing magazines that feature patterns in the midsection. Most patterns come with simple, easily-followed step-by-step instructions. Follow them meticulously, but not religiously. If you know what you are doing, patterns can be modified accordingly.

Once you have acquired the right pattern, you need to obtain the materials for the dress. Patterns generally have recommendations on what fabrics are suitable for the dress in question. Some fabrics have characteristics that make them more difficult to handle and sew, and thus are not suitable for inexperienced seamstresses.

Note also that most prom dress fabrics and materials cannot be machine washed, but need dry-cleaning. Buy more fabric than recommended in the pattern instructions just in case. You might also want to make an extra item from the same material even if nothing goes wrong the first time.

After carefully familiarizing yourself with the instructions, you may begin cutting out the pattern pieces needed. One option is to cut straight from the patterns, or you can copy them to a separate sheet so that the original patterns can be re-used, borrowed or perhaps sold to someone afterwards.

Once you have the pattern pieces cut, you place them on the fabric. Place the material on a clean, level surface to avoid any mishaps. After this, pin the pattern pieces on the fabric. You could sketch out the patterns on the fabric. By doing this, the cutting of the fabric becomes easier and more manageable. After you have cut all the items, begin sewing according to instructions.

Funerals

The universal dress code for funerals is something smart, understated and black. However, there is more to it. In addition, women's funeral wear should be modest but dressy, tasteful and yet somber, and naturally, appropriate for the season. Your relationship with the deceased also affects your attire.

All in all, your attire should not divert the attention away from the fact that the attendants have gathered to mourn, and therefore it is important to plan your outfit in advance and make necessary purchases.

A black shift dress and a matching suit jacket or a blazer makes a good outfit if this is your family member's funeral. A blouse and a skirt are also acceptable for this occasion. In warmer climate, a short sleeved fitted dress works just as well.

Sleeveless or strapless dresses, however, should be avoided on their own. If you plan to wear a black sleeveless or strapless dress, cover your shoulders with a jacket, a coat or a wrap. Make sure you co-ordinate your shoes and bag with the attire, and take weather conditions in to consideration.

A black veil is no longer a must, but weather permitting you might want one. Alternatively, you could choose a dark pill hat with added veil detail in the front. For close family funerals, head-to-toe black is recommended.

If the funeral is a friend or family funeral, navy blue, gray or violet are acceptable colors to be added to the attire. Although bright colors should be avoided, a white blouse or shirt can be worn with otherwise darker skirt and jacket or blazer.

In an unexpected funeral, your most conservative outfit will do if you don't already have traditional funeral attire selected. Short skirts and low necklines should always be avoided at funerals.

Graduation Parties

First thing to establish is the nature of the graduation party you have been invited to. Where will the party happen? A small, casual party at a restaurant is a completely different affair to a ballroom event, and so is a barbeque at a family member's backyard.

Generally, graduation parties range from very casual to more formal. There is no set universal standard for the graduation party guests. It is best to use common sense. For those of you, who will be hosting a graduation party, make sure you include details on the invitation regarding the type of event and the dress code.

If a specific dress code is not specified on the invitation, ring up the graduate and ask for more information while simultaneously RSVP: in the event itself. Another option is to get in touch with other people you know are also attending. If you have any idea who is coming, that is. You could coordinate or de-code the dress code among yourself.

This way, you'll at least have some people who are equally dressed as you. Additionally, this might save you the embarrassment of wearing an identical outfit with your friend. Sometimes, these things happen.

If you are the graduate, keep in mind that you will be wearing a cap and gown over your attire. At least this is customary in most countries. General rule of thumb is that you should wear something more formal than jeans and flip-flops.

A casual dress or a nice blouse and smart trousers should do the trick. Perhaps this is the chance for you to obtain that all-essential little black dress. If you feel comfortable in more bold and vivid colors, this is wholeheartedly recommended and not a tad inappropriate, just coordinate your colors with cap and gown to avoid huge clashes.

When considering footwear, take into consideration the location and length of event. Black pumps will work, but you might feel uncomfortable standing up in stilettos or killer heels for long times, and it could be embarrassing to look like your feet are killing you in front of everyone.

If you are a family member or a parent of the graduate, you'll want to dress up nicely as well. Not only your son, daughter or other family member will be the center of focus, but you'll appear in many photographs as well.

As the graduate, the location aspect goes for you as well. Will you be outside in the sun? Perhaps a hat could be added on to the attire to avoid sun strokes. Is it going to be rainy or chilly? Weather conditions need to be considered when putting together the outfit. For photographic purposes, you might want to coordinate with the graduate's gown so that clashes are avoided. Crazy patterns might be a tad risky, too.

What to Wear to Dates?

Dates can be just as tricky as job interviews attire wise. These two occasions have other similarities as well: it is the first impression that carries a lot of weight. Follow these tips on what to wear, and focus on stressing out on the other codes of behavior that might make or break the date night.

You want to give the impression that you're sassy, sexy and fun. Consider not revealing too much skin or in a provocative manner, as this will surely not spell out sexy but sends out an entirely unintended message.

It can be complicated on deciding whether you're simply showing off your best bits, or too provocative. You are essentially the best judge of that – do you feel comfortable and good-looking, or a stripper in your own standards?

A suitable, sober outfit could for example consist of a fancier silk shirt or blouse coupled with a pencil skirt, or more casual pair of jeans. If – perhaps after the first date – you get together in a casual setting, ditch the silk blouse and wear something you would in any casual occasion, a cardigan, perhaps?

Hair and make-up on first date is ideally natural, but add on some glamor to impress. Easiest way of determining what is chic enough is to compare your hair and makeup to office standards. Would you feel a bit too dressed up in this hairdo and that make-up, if you went to work in it on Monday morning?

If you are unsure what you will be doing for your date, don't panic. Calmly approach your closet and pick up the little black dress of yours. This old favorite will be dressy enough for fancier occasions, but not completely out of place in a less formal setting.

What if it all turns out to be okay and you eventually meet his or her parents, friends, colleagues, in fact anyone close to him? Try and remain natural at these events: natural in attire, make-up and behavior.

Clubbing with the Girls

Big nights out require attires that match the evening. It is your personal experience, taste and dress codes that ultimately determine what to wear at specific clubs. Here, we will not try to force everyone into the same mold by defining what is most suitable to wear on a night out. Rather, we have gathered some tips that might help you in dressing up and looking your best.

What does it mean in practice if the club has a casual dress code? Jeans and flip-flops? Not to worry, casual dress code at clubs allows you to feel comfortable if you're just heading out to dance the night away with your girlfriends. At the same time, it doesn't prevent you to dress up flamboyantly if you wish to come across new people or meet up with a dream date.

You could for example throw on skinny jeans and a more festive top — perhaps sleeveless or strapless. Nothing wrong with curve-accentuating brightly colored dresses either. Show off as much skin as you desire and can comfortably do.

If moving about is difficult because you feel you're about to flash, then you are definitely in the wrong outfit and all elegance is lost. We want to stand out, but not because of something embarrassing we did. Club nights are a good testing ground for new fashions and a bit more eclectic style choices.

Make-up should be darker than in the office, mainly because of the lighting. Emphasize one key feature with your make-up, for example if you highlight your lips then go easy on the eyes and vice versa.

Your trusted little black dress could easily be worn in clubs without the fear of overdressing. Most women want to impress and catch attention at clubs, so a little black dress is as good as a choice of attire as any other.

As per usual, accessorizing your cocktail dress is the key here. Killer heels and statement jewelry will personalize and differentiate your little black number from the little black number you just wore to work.

When it comes to shoes, they are of essence when wearing your cocktail dress out to a club. Your shoes ought to highlight the fact that you are sassy, chic and out to have fun. Go for example with stilettos, which will elongate your legs and create the illusion of slimmer legs. Alternatively, you could put on a pair of heels that have sparks, studs or sequins that will get the party started.

Your handbag should also reflect the fact that you are out and about, having a good time. Although a tote bag doubles as a handbag and briefcase, opt for a less office-y look and go for a cute clutch bag instead.

Will your essentials – cash and lipstick – fit in? Then it's perfect. Your handbag should be more colorful and bold to bring in some life to your otherwise black and simple cocktail dress.

As far as the jewelry goes, a statement piece is a must. Keep in mind that all of your jewelry – earrings, rings, bracelets and necklaces – needn't be over the top. One chunky, bold and eye catching piece of jewelry will do the trick on its own. If you wear all kinds of chunky gold all over, you'll end up looking like a rap star and not an elegant woman letting her hair down.

Another office item that could be easily transformed into club wear is the pencil skirt. If you are heading out straight from work, transforming a pencil skirt based attire from business to another kind of business is fairly easy.

Just remember the tricks applied to cocktail dress. Add stilettos and a statement jewelry piece likes dangling earrings to begin with. For a rocker chick look, add on a band t-shirt. If that doesn't sound like your cup of tea, opt for a sexy blouse.

If you and your pals are meeting up in a bar instead of dancing yourselves silly in a club, you could wear something a bit more relaxed. Naturally, you want to look your best, however. Again, it might be easy to stand out too much by overdressing, which can leave you feeling uncomfortable.

If the bar you are heading to is one that you frequently visit, you probably already have a good idea what to wear and not feel out of place. It might be trickier in case this is a new spot for you and your girlfriends.

Essentially, you will know in advance whether the place is a classy upscale place or a sports bar. In the so-called dive bars or dingier pubs, you might want to leave your best clothes at home and focus on being comfortable and drunk.

Sports bars usually have a comfortable, relaxed and a casual crowd, so jeans will do just fine. Mid-scale bars or concept bars that normally have after work happy hours should be approached looking like you've just finished at the office.

Upscale, roof top or hotel bars require more formal attire and basically, you should wear your best. Stilettos and designer bags go far in here.

Carnivals and Fancy Dress Parties

Carnivals as well as fancy dress parties are great occasions of going wild and throwing on an outfit that you would not normally get caught in. Carnival dresses most often consist of sequins, feathers and show quite a bit of skin.

Of course, there are variations depending on the country and the nature of the carnival. Check out article titled Carnival Costumes up on www.escapade.co.uk webpage for further information. We will go through here some of their suggestions on carnival attires and top carnival destinations.

In Roman Carnevale at the Pont St. Martin, chariot races take place alongside burning of a devil statue. Bring your nyph or toga costumes with you, as this is the 'dress code' in the crowd. See the next chapter on period costumes for advice on how to fashion and don a toga true Roman Empire style. Livigno Carnevale that is celebrated by the Alps and Swiss border culminates in a fancy dress ball. The next chapter will also offer advice on fancy dress occasions.

Nice Carnival in France is one of the biggest festivals in the world and set to a particular theme every year. There will be a parade and the French dress up in *deguisement,* or fancy dress for the occasion. Parisian Carnival takes place on late February, and it is a traditional Mardi Gras celebration. Attendants and partygoers dress up in traditional carnival costumes. Mardi Gras outfits can contain colorful beads, wigs, hats and masks.

Sitges Carnival in Barcelona, Spain is normally held at the beginning of February and lasting until mid-February. According to Escapade article, around 250,000 revelers show up for the event. For this occasion, throw on a disfraz or disfraced para carnaval – a drag dress or a carnival fancy dress. Dressing up in drag isn't a possibility that creeps up every day! Remember masks for Sitges Carnival.

Other fancy dress carnivals take place for example in Portuguese towns of Ovar, Loures, Podence, Louié, Sesimbra and Torres Verdas. Fantasy Fest in Key West, Florida in the United States lasts for ten days and ends with a huge themed costume extravaganza.

Your attire could be a fairy-tale princess, a famous movie star or a cartoon character. Whatever you opt for, don't underdress for the carnival. If ever, now is the time to add sparkle, sequins, and feathers, anything unusual and outrageous that you normally wouldn't dare to sport in public.

Fastelavn in Denmark begins on Monday before Ash Wednesday, and is a Danish version of Halloween party. This is because youngsters run around in costumes and get treats, but adults are not entirely encouraged to take part in celebrations donning a spooky outfit.

Polish carnival in February also has a similar feel to Halloween and is celebrated on the last day before lent. Is one ever too old to be a sexy vampire, a hot zombie nurse or sensual Cat Woman? The answer in our books is, 'no'.

The most famous of all the carnivals take place in Rio de Janeiro, Brazil and begin in February. The carnival has become known around the world for its outstanding festivity and music, as well as the stunning costumes on the revelers.

Strict dress codes do not exist, but you should keep in mind a few unwritten rules if attending carnival in Rio. Skimpier options are not frowned upon; Brazilians are comfortable in their skin.

If you feel comfortable in shorts, miniskirts and short tops, you can easily wear them. Keep in mind the weather conditions. It is bound to be hot, and the temper will rise amongst the crowded parts.

Sandals or flip flops are acceptable footwear. If you participate in any of the performances, you will be required to wear the over-the-top costumes that dancers wear. This same costume can be kept on in street parties later, in the Scala balls or pretty much anywhere. It will not create unwanted attention outside the parade.

Fancy dress parties are a really good occasion to let loose and go wild with outfits. Dressing up could take place in Halloween, for instance. Fancy dress parties are a fun option even for adult birthdays or just a good excuse of getting together with friends and going silly.

You could either arrange a themed fancy dress party – such as the always popular toga party – or let the guests choose for themselves. Need inspiration for fancy dress parties? Look no further.

Let us start with some historical looks. What should a woman wear, if she wants to present herself in the Roman period attire at a fancy dress party? Roman items are quite simple to make at home, and with the right kind of hairdos and accessories are a good, easily constructed look for a fancy dress party.

Tunics or togas work fine, attach them at the sides with broaches or buttons. The fabric flows freely over the body. You might want to add a little sass for modern occasions with a more fitted cut. It's up to you, whether you want to go for authenticity or accentuation.

Toga was common clothing both in Rome and Ancient Greece, actually. Togas could be worn by both genders, so mixed sex toga parties shouldn't offend anyone's sense of authenticity. Togas are also noteworthy Roman artifacts in a sense that they did not reflect social rank initially.

How to wear the toga properly? The fabric is first placed over the left shoulder, and part of it is left hanging loose in the front. Toga is then passed around the back from the shoulder and under right arm. Finally, throw the fabric over left shoulder. Roman footwear for ladies ought to be sandals, if the weather permits them.

Old Hollywood is another good theme that generates a communal feel at the party and immediately feeds guests imagination while still allowing people to express their individuality.

For Old Hollywood parties, you could either dress up as a cinema icon from the past – think for example Marilyn Monroe in that famous, flowy and white halter neck summer dress or Audrey Hepburn in her signature black cocktail dress with glamorous diamonds. Fancy dress costume stores normally carry a good range of outfits that fit the cinema theme.

One option that could be worn again and again is European aristocrat from the past. This costume fit for a queen could either be purchased or tailor made. To get the right look, you need a period dress, possibly a wig depending on the era you are going for with your dress, careful make up and accessories that were fashionable once upon a time.

A good source for researching this topic is educational costume history websites. For our purposes here, I've paraphrased material from Scott R. Robinson's page up on http://www.cwu.edu/~robinsos/. Robinson himself is a theatre costume designer and a professor of theatre arts.

Let's begin with Renaissance looks fit for a queen. Renaissance as a period is only fifty years long and it dates from 1450 to 1500. During this period, excessiveness is the key word. This new ideal in fashion took wind underneath its wings. However, there are regional variations on how excessiveness was incorporated into clothing.

Northern European countries distorted the 'naturalness' by favoring padded sleeves, doublets and stockings. The idea behind excessive was to make improvements to the natural silhouette, which is not very 'far out' or alien to modern day fashions actually.

Large puffs were placed at the head, shoulders, and thighs. Smaller puffs were put over chest, back, arms, legs and feet. Consider adding a 'stomacher' to your costume – by 'stomacher' we mean an ornamental or additional padding in the bodice.

Feathers are essential decorative elements when combining a true Renaissance costume. They were used in wide-brimmed hats, for instance, but could be sticked on to any imaginable garment.

Panel and conjoined elements are also present in other garments. It was typical at the time for the fabric of the garment to feature slits, through which a different fabric appeared. Sometimes it was the plain, white underclothing that was revealed through slits.

When it comes to head pieces and hairstyles, women of the Renaissance covered their heads with low-crowned hats. One notable element in Renaissance costume is kennel or gable headdresses, and a Renaissance princess at fancy dress parties you should simply don one.

In these headdresses, a piece covers the front part of the head and ears. A veil covers rest of the head. Note that no hair was visible in formal attire. The front 'roll' of this was usually velvet. The kennel contained a stiff plane wrapped in rich material and the cap at the back joined the bag-like kennel.

Elizabethan period dates from 1550 to 1625.Materials were plain-colored and brocaded, and jewel use increased. Perhaps this era could be labeled as the definite period of collars. Typically, Elizabethan collars were starched very high up using many ruffles. Take for example wisk – a standing, fan shaped wired collar. Again, as is typical for fashion, the beauty ideals of the day affected and influenced the structure of the garments and trends. What was considered beautiful in Elizabethan times, then? Long waists, long legs and small heads. A more slender look overtook the previously fashionable and idealized squarish silhouette. Huge hips were sought after, and thus the hoop appeared.

Aside the hoops worn under skirts, perhaps a stuffed roll tied around waist was added for that little bit of extra lift. These rolls under skirts are called bolsters, and perhaps hoops under an Elizabethan fancy dress will impair your mobility. Now, we don't want to stand still in such a festive event, so perhaps only bolsters will do the trick. Second usable and authentic way of creating volume under skirt is layers and layers of petticoats.

Women wore their hair drawn away from the ears and the temple was fluffed. Apparently, the widow's peak, or a V-shaped peak in the middle of hairline was a fashionable detail. Blonde and red hair colors were fashionable. Hair was either dyed or bleached, but wearing a wig was also an option.

The Restoration period began in 1660 and ended in 1700. Next, we will focus on the Restoration costume and how the style of the day might be used in fancy dress occasions. More elaborate and excessive fashion returned. For example, it was a common practice to attach ornamental and decorative curls, ribbons, puff, flounces and feathers wherever imaginable. Both in women's and men's fashion stiffness and smart elegance of the prior era began re-emerging.

Collars were higher and wider, reaching across the shoulders. Necklines were low, wide, and dropped on the shoulders. Underdress was worn with another garment on top, and the bodice and skirt were attached. This was a financial and societal barrier, as poorer women apparently could not afford attached skirts and bodices. So, common women could be identified from mix matched bodices and skirts. Hemlines were still long, but toes could be visible.

Manteau gowns originate from the period of Louis XIV, The Sun King of France. In this era, the overskirt is looped back and held in place with ribbon bows. An underskirt of manteau is often a taffeta. You will recognize manteau from the 'train' carried over left arm – expect when in presence of royalty. There is a fun fact to keep in mind at fancy dress occasions.

Accessory wise, apron is the most notable addition to fashionable costumes. Cannons, or bunches of ribbons, wore worn around the knee. Ringlets still remained fashionable in women's hair do's, but they were gathered in the back of the head. Smaller ringlets, wisps of hair, were left around the face. Pearls or nosegays could be incorporated into the hair-do of the Restoration period. White caps were worn still in Europe and in the colonies in North America.

Color schemes varied from France to colonies: whereas in English court and Versailles deep-toned velvet and light colored satin prevailed, whereas in Colonial fashion bright-hued garments prevailed. During this period, red, blue, yellow and green were bravely combined.

France became the dictator of new styles in this eighteenth century. The key elements of 18th century styles were wigs, powdered hair, porcelain-complexions, slender bodices, distended skirts, wide coat-tails, clocked silk stockings, red-heeled shoes, flowers, ribbons and lace. However, later in the course of the eighteenth century 'naturalness' became vogue and the hair styles did not require masses of powder any longer.

In the early 18th century, women wore masculine periwigs but their wigs parted in the middle. The further the time went, the bigger the hair became. It is said that a fashionable lady's wig was adjusted by a hairdressers standing on ladders. Perhaps going to such lengths are not the most functional or practical when it comes to your fancy dress attire, but it would certainly catch other guest's attention. This Pompadour hair-do's is normally associated with French court and can be further decorated with birds or toys, even.

Ideally the upper body of women was slim, tight and long-waisted. Bodices reflected this and soon became corset shape. In 18th century, hoops became fashionable again. Fronts of the corsets could be highly decorated, and these fronts were known as plastrons.

During the nineteenth century necklines rose higher and if the necklines were dropped about the shoulder lines, ruffs covered the neck. Corsets were worn again and waist emphasized with possibly a belt with a large buckle. Short sleeves were puffed at the top. Long sleeves were of leg-o-mutton shape.

Hairstyle was normally a smooth arrangement and parted in the middle. Ringlets or loops framed the face. Cap became an acceptable accessory used together with house dress. In the evenings, caps gave room to turbans that accompanied evening gowns. Bonnets and hats were worn for day or night time outdoor activities. Women's colors of these periods were restricted to raised, celestial, lapis blue, cream, yellow, pale green, dove and lavender gray. Pastel colors were reserved for children's clothing. Undergarments comprised of chemise, corset and various petticoats.

For chilly fancy dress affairs, a dolman could be added on to the Crinoline attire. Dolman is a three-quarter length wrap normally made of brocade, silk, or woolen material. Dolman's sleeves are cut in one with the body. Black or colored silks were used to tie up the hair that was in a knot in the back of the head. Hair was either curled in ringlets, or braided about the head. Popular colors at the beginning of these periods were pastels and white when it came to evening gowns. Day wear could be lavender, lilac, tan, silver-gray, gray-green and silver blue, for example.

Later on, women began wearing darker colors again. For instance, red, blue, crimson, maroon, brown, dark green, purple, plum, magenta and violet were in fashion.

One key element that differentiates the end of nineteenth century from its predecessors was the standardization of clothing. In 1860s, hips became central in beauty ideals dictating the female body shape. Consequently, women with lesser hips began enhancing their lower half of the body with the aid of fashion and clothing. Corseting hips became a standard practice. High-heeled shoes known as 'Grecian Bends' emphasized a curving rear.

The Victorian corset raised high in the front to push up the bust, and curved out over the abdomen and hips. As professor Robinson points out, corsets of the day pressed firmly upon ribs, diaphragm and internal organs. This, as you can imagine, is very painful.

Indeed, Victorian corsets have been considered oppressing the women. Liberation from the corsets altogether began at the beginning of the twentieth century. Perhaps, for fancy dress occasions the Victorian corset is too hard core and certainly will not make you comfortable and ready to unwind in a social setting.

By far, black was the most popular color amongst women during Bustle period. However, women could freely wear any colors at that time. There were no strict restrictions based on social status or any other factor, and paradoxically at the time as any color could have been worn, the simple black became the option women really went for.

Our chapter on eighteenth century costume ends with the fin-de-siécle period consisting of the last decade of the century. Women in this 'dandy' period wore a more comfortable dress with the pendulum swung back. Sleeves suddenly became massive again: they were about the size of a balloon and contained enough fabric for a whole dress. Skirt spread from eighteen inch wasp-waist to the ground.

Chesterfields appeared. These are fitted dress overcoats with hidden buttons and a velvet collar. Women's tops became detached from the skirt. The focal point shifted from shoulders to the front. Gibson Girls were blouses with a single pleat that stretched from shoulder to shoulder and also front to back.

In women's shoes, toothpick toes and high heels were the style of the day. The shoes narrowed towards the toe, and the heels were considerably higher than ever before. Hats tended to be smaller than in previous times.

Women's hair do's consisted of backcomb from the forehead. The hair was knotted on top with a pompadour. The French Twist was popular in the last decade of the century. This hairstyle fits modern, classy women as well so consider donning one to a fancy dress party if you are going for the fin-de-siecle look.

Here we reach again the beginning of the twentieth century fashions, where this book began initially. We have covered some wide ranging fields, and hopefully you, the reader, go out and play with the acquired knowledge, tips and inspiration.